THE CAMOUFLAGED HEART

SUSIE GUCKIN

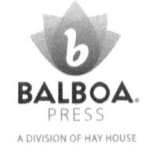

BALBOA.
PRESS

A DIVISION OF HAY HOUSE

Balboa Press books may be ordered through booksellers or by contacting:

Balboa Press
A Division of Hay House
1663 Liberty Drive
Bloomington, IN 47403
www.balboapress.com
1 (877) 407-4847

Print information available on the last page.

ISBN: 978-1-5043-3031-2 (sc)
ISBN: 978-1-5043-3033-6 (hc)
ISBN: 978-1-5043-3032-9 (e)

Library of Congress Control Number: 2015904796

Balboa Press rev. date: 04/14/2015

CONTENTS

Dedication.. vii

About the Author ix

Introduction xi

Preface xiii

Chapter 1   How It All Began 1

Chapter 2   Early Symptoms and Another
            Accident 4

Chapter 3   Less Obvious Symptoms 10

Chapter 4   Symptom Specifics 18

Chapter 5   Overcoming Obstacles 24

Chapter 6   Seeking Help... 36

Chapter 7   My Greatest Teachers 41

Chapter 8   The Process.. 48

Chapter 9   Fear As Fuel 52

Chapter 10 Dealing With Fears And Changed
            Relationships 59
Chapter 11 Experiencing Life Through New
            Eyes.. 68
Chapter 12 A Remarkable Coincidence................. 73
Chapter 13 The Camouflaged Heart...................... 76
Chapter 14 Seeds of Service 79

Acknowledgements 85

DEDICATION

To the many brave men and women
who have served our country and
know the peril of PTSD and TBI.

Thank you for all that you continue to teach
each of us about courage and recovery.

ABOUT THE AUTHOR

Susie Guckin is a "Warriors at Ease" certified meditation teacher with advanced training in military combat stress, trauma, post-traumatic stress, and resiliency. She is also a McLean Meditation Institute certified meditation teacher with training in stress reduction and stress management, as well as, a Reiki II practitioner. She is the owner of "Peaceful Warriors" offering trauma-sensitive meditation and energy work at the Jersey Shore.

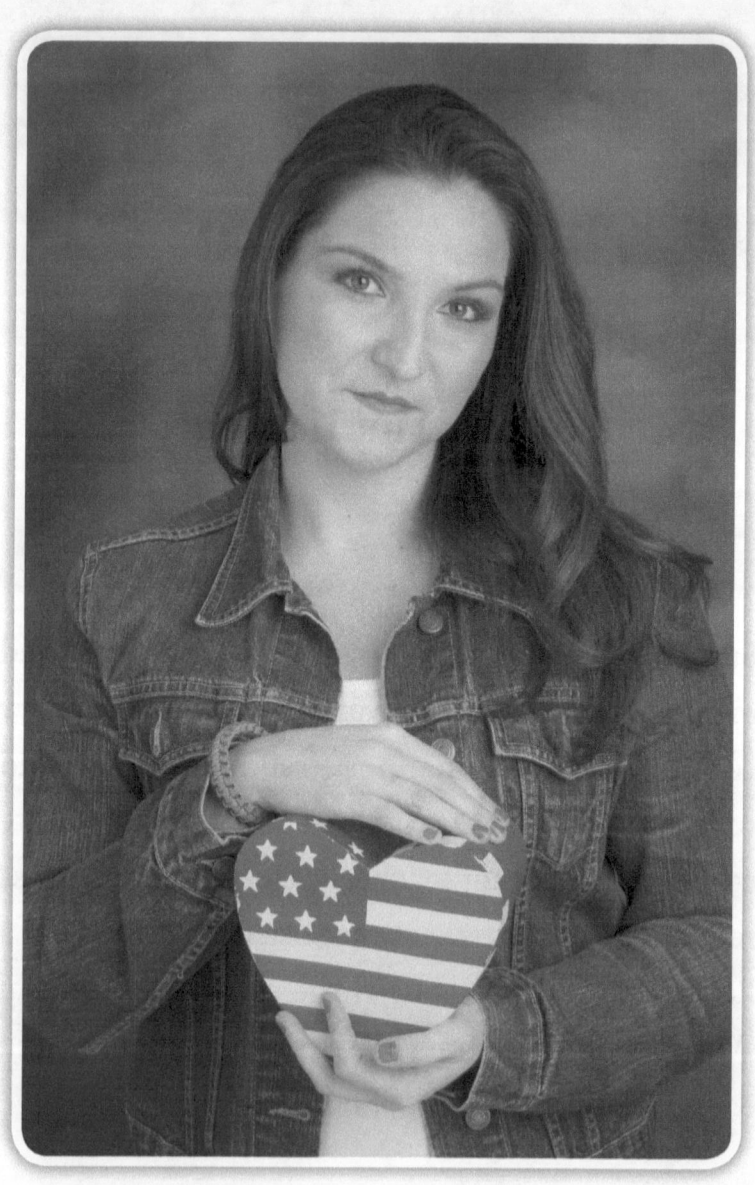

INTRODUCTION

I once met with a military chaplain who was very kind to me. He said, "Susie, you have infiltrated a brotherhood that doesn't trust anyone except each other. You are what we call a "wounded healer." A wounded healer is someone who has come through trauma and survived to tell the tale of how they recovered as a means to help others. I didn't understand the statement he made at the time, but I can clearly see what he meant by it. I have been in the "trenches" of injury, self-defeat, post-traumatic stress (PTSD), and traumatic brain injury (TBI) from the car accidents I experienced. The soldiers I have befriended along my path of recovery from my injuries told me it doesn't matter whether I have ever been to war or if I have ever served in the military. They weren't interested in judging my experience or looking at how I got hurt, just that I somehow understood how they were feeling from the inside out. I know trauma and I know PTSD. With that, I have crawled out of the "trenches" and am extending my hand to the others who are trying to climb their way out towards recovery too.

If you know someone who suffers from TBI or PTSD, or maybe you are the one suffering from their impact on your life, this story is for you. I challenge you to believe that life isn't about suffering. It's about growth. Growing from our experiences whether they appear to be good or bad, is all part of living our lives. Consider that maybe our trauma is part of our evolution as a human being, not the breaking down of a human being.

PREFACE

I come from a family with a history of military service in several branches of the United States military. My father was a drill instructor at Fort Dix during the Vietnam Era. My parents lived on post, where my father was eventually medically retired. My appreciation for the military was modeled by my mother, and my appreciation for the plight of soldiers and other military personnel comes from my own experiences with trauma and post-traumatic stress, as well as nine years of volunteering with soldiers at the same base my parents had lived on. I am the owner of "Peaceful Warriors", which offers trauma-sensitive meditation and energy work for the benefit of stress reduction, stress management, and relaxation. I became interested in meditation after many years of suffering with the symptoms of PTSD and TBI due to two car accidents at age twenty. Meditation has created a sense of solace, centeredness, control, and normalcy in my life. My journey led me to Joint Base McGuire-Dix-Lakehurst in New Jersey, where I became a volunteer with the USO and eventually was introduced to the medical hold, formerly known as the Warrior Transition Unit (WTU). While volunteering at the WTU over a period of nine years, I was in the company of soldiers and other military personnel who suffered many of the same kinds of symptoms I had. The common ground I found led me to seek out ways of overcoming the symptoms that seemed to plague all people with PTSD, whether it was related to war, accidents, abuse, or injury.

This put me on the path to wanting to offer methods of relaxation to the soldiers and others who have been suffering with symptoms of PTSD and trauma, so I took the steps necessary to become a certified meditation teacher. I believe that when you plant seeds of hope through meditation and energy work, they will grow for each person in their own way and in their own time, leading people to regain a sense of who they are beyond their symptoms.

My earlier path began with a degree in music education from the College of New Jersey. Since my graduation twelve years ago, I have worked as a band and orchestra director in a public school. Through my experiences as a public school music teacher and private music instructor, I have taught children of varying needs and abilities, as well as, medical and psychological conditions. It seemed this was a natural first step in learning how to use compassionate teaching to help others.

During my employment with the school district, I have developed a positive relationship with the local military base's community outreach program. The military community outreach program connected military personnel with the community to draw awareness and education about the great service that military members provide for New Jersey, the United States, and the world beyond simply preparing for war.

I am also a member of the Eastern Wind Symphony of Princeton, New Jersey. I have been a member of the wind symphony, playing clarinet, for ten years, completing performances most recently at Carnegie Hall in March of 2013, Richardson Auditorium of Princeton University 2014/2015, and two previous performances at the "John F. Kennedy Center for the Performing Arts", Washington, D.C., and Patriot's Theater at the War Memorial, Trenton, NJ. During the first performance at the Kennedy Center for the *National Memorial Day Choral Festival in 2008*, late actor and World War II Veteran Mickey Rooney was in attendance. He was awarded a commendation and letter of appreciation signed by the Secretary of the Army and the Army Chief of Staff, recognizing his dedication and support of soldiers. The performance at Carnegie Hall for the *Eastern Wind Symphony Symphonic Gala* in 2013, had in attendance two of the last surviving Tuskegee Airmen, as one of the pieces performed was originally commissioned in honor of the Tuskegee Airmen by the United States Air Force Band. It was then commissioned for wind ensemble by the Eastern Wind Symphony for the Carnegie Hall world premier performance. The culmination of these tremendous experiences has been shaped through my trauma and my recovery. It is these experiences that have made telling this story so important for the good of others. I can only hope that what I have been encouraged to share has the ability to help others on their own personal journey of recovery. I am inspired by my experiences and continue to make music, healing, and service to others part of my life each day.

CHAPTER 1

HOW IT ALL BEGAN

We are often so busy surviving that we are unaware
of how fragile life is and how quickly a traumatic
event can alter our very existence. I was twenty years
old when I was in two car accidents that happened
fairly close together. These accidents changed my
life tremendously. As I share with you my journey
over the past fourteen years through traumatic brain
injury and post-traumatic stress, you will be able to
see not only the emotional and mental unraveling of
a person, but also that person's amazing evolution

through trauma. The first car accident seemed relatively simple and uneventful. A deer ran into the driver's-side front end of my car. The car was damaged, but it was nothing tragic. It was in drivable condition from the accident and so I returned home. I was shaken, but overall I was fine. There wasn't a scratch on me. The next day I played in a concert. At the time I was a music student, aspiring to be a music teacher. My lifelong passion to teach music and to work with children will become an important part of this story as it unfolds. My mother attended my concert that day, as she always did. When we arrived back at my apartment, I was feeling fatigued and drained, and I had a bit of a headache. I promised my mother that I was okay, and she returned home. The next morning she called me, and my speech was slurred. Although I was disoriented, I promised her again that I was fine. She knew better. My mother came right over and took me to the hospital. The triage nurses proceeded to ask the usual barrage of questions, only one of which—"What's your name?"—was I able to answer correctly. I could not provide my birthdate, my address, my social security number, or the day of the week. Wishing they would save their questions for someone who cared, I became increasingly angry and belligerent at their prodding. It felt as if my personal files were in my mind; I knew that I knew the answers, but for some reason I couldn't access the file, and the nurses were making it worse. I was taken in for a brain scan. While I was in radiology for the procedure, I threw up and passed out. The doctors diagnosed me with a concussion and told me to follow up with my primary-care doctor.

CHAPTER 2

EARLY SYMPTOMS AND ANOTHER ACCIDENT

There is a standard procedure in place for the care of a concussion. The primary care doctor knew exactly what to tell me to do at the time. My slurred speech, disorientation, and short-term memory impairment was pretty standard for a concussion. But several other symptoms showed up as well. I had slowed motor skills and coordination, as well as some sensitivity to sound and light. My doctor instructed me to take a couple weeks off from my college courses to rest at home. She told me to limit physical activity and to avoid doing anything that would tax my brain—including watching television, reading, and playing video games. For someone who had no recollection of hitting her head, this was a long list of symptoms and orders to follow. It was all rather baffling. But I felt that if I wanted to get better and get back to school, then I had to do everything the doctor told me to do. Besides, my focus was very limited; I felt far from prepared to do any of the activities that the doctor prohibited. I was extremely tired all the time. One moment I would be talking to someone, and the next I would fall asleep. My brain was trying to repair itself through rest, and I was doing everything in my power to support it.

Two months later I went back to school. I wasn't quite operating on all cylinders, but I was functioning and glad to be back. My motor skills were a bit slowed, but again, it was nothing that was going to get in my way for long. Reading and other tasks were also a bit difficult, but the doctor assured me that all of these symptoms would improve over time.

One evening, after dark, just two months after the first accident, I was driving back to school after a visit with my mother, and I was in another accident. I was traveling on a highway at about 65 to 70 miles per hour when there was a buckling noise. The hood came unlatched, flew up over the windshield, and broke the front end frame of the car where the hood attached to the body of the car. The force of the hood unlatching sent the car careening off the road. The hood had been damaged in the first accident, but it hadn't needed to be fully replaced. Instead, it had been banged out and reset. There was a small space on the driver's side where the force of the wind could have ripped the hood from the latch. I don't recall the accident—which is something I will discuss later— but at the time I told the state trooper that there had been a Mack truck to my right, and my car had pulled off to the right. I didn't know how I had ended up to the left, in the center median. The trooper couldn't believe that I was alive, without a single physical scratch. I had survived two freak accidents in a very short span of time.

It's known that if you have one head injury, you have one set of problems, as well as one set of orders to follow in your care and recovery. It is also known that head injuries are cumulative. The second injury creates a much more extreme set of problems than the first. My blurred vision was more intense than it had been after the first accident. The light and sound sensitivity were also stronger. I squinted often and felt very irritated by sunlight or any other bright light. I wanted everything to be dim. The best way that I can describe the sound sensitivity is that everything felt amplified, as if there were two megaphones up to my ears. Beeping noises were the worst, and crowded places were a nightmare. My motor-skill issues were now more pronounced. Unable to think through coordinated movements, I found myself dropping things, tripping over my own feet, and overall not feeling in control of my own body. The short-term memory loss returned with a vengeance. I was having difficulty remembering anything from one minute to the next. You could have a conversation with me, and two seconds later I wouldn't remember that you were even in the same room with me. You could call me five times in one day, and I would tell you each time that I hadn't heard from you in ages. I became lost in time and unsure of which hour it was—or sometimes even *what* an hour was. My doctor said that because I had had two head injuries so close together, my recovery time could be more than doubled. She recommended that I consider dropping out of school. At the sound of that, I panicked, cried, and said, "No!" Was I really to believe that I couldn't get better? That I would have to give up everything I had worked for because of two accidents that I couldn't have prevented? I just wouldn't hear of it. I didn't know how long it would take me to get better, but I wasn't going to give up on school. At that, we contacted my professors and told them what had happened. They agreed to "play it by ear" and hold my grades as incomplete until after the New Year, which was two months away.

I can't say that I was truly ready when I returned to school that January. I had spent the months leading up to that following the recommendations that the doctor had given me to rest as much as possible. I was still experiencing a lot of deficiencies. I was not allowed to drive, so I had to rely on friends to get from one place to another. My ability to concentrate was terribly compromised, and it was very frustrating. Again, it was as if my brain held files that just wouldn't open. I had trouble decoding words. I would see letters but not understand the word that they formed. I would stare and stare, trying to make sense of them, playing instruments was a challenge because my ability to read music was impaired, and my fingers felt like they had lead weights in them. No matter how hard I tried, they didn't move as fast as everyone else's.

Not every symptom of a head injury is something that jumps right out at you. Some take time to recognize and decode. For me, an impaired sense of direction was one of those. Until you are in a position where you must rely on your internal compass, you won't realize it's not working. When I had to navigate campus alone, I found myself getting lost in familiar places. I would stare at buildings as if I had never seen them before. I was too embarrassed to ask people nearby for help, and I couldn't remember where my friends lived on campus. Again, that file in my brain just wasn't opening. I didn't have access. Thank God for cell phones with automatic dialing. I would call my mother, and she would tell me where to go. One evening I actually had to call a cab to get home—and it's a good thing I had my address written down, or it would have been one long taxi ride.

CHAPTER 3

LESS OBVIOUS SYMPTOMS

I graduated from college with a degree in music. I had fought my way through the confusing and frustrating physical symptoms of my injuries that had caused motor skill impairments, headaches, coordination problems, and impaired vision. I was now embarking on a new job as a teacher in a very good school district. Remarkably, I had gone on the interview at the prompting of a former teacher of mine. He always had known what was best for me, and this time had been no different. After my very first interview, I had gotten the job—and the interviewers had said that there was something special about me. This had meant the world to me after all that I had been through—and was still going through. I was willing to put my all into succeeding.

Shortly after successfully completing my interview, I moved into my own apartment in a town nearby to the school district I was to be teaching in. It was a beautiful apartment on the second floor of a Victorian home. It had a screened-in porch on the top floor and a sweet, charming energy. It was only when I was truly on my own that I started to discover the deeper damage that my head injuries had done. Performing daily tasks was unusually difficult. I would wake up in the morning, sit on the edge of the bed, and wonder what I was supposed to do first. Then, still unsure of what was supposed to happen, I would walk into the kitchen, into the bathroom, and then back into the bedroom. The file was there, but again, I was unable to access it. I felt anxious, upset, and pressured by my confusion. I would then hurriedly throw on some clothes and run out the door. Halfway to my destination, I would realize that I hadn't taken my asthma medicine or made myself a lunch. It was a very defeating feeling.

In the wintertime, more symptoms began to emerge. My brain's wiring for the sense and feel of temperature was not working properly. I would run down the stairs to leave in the morning, see frost, and tell myself that frost meant that it must be cold. Then I would look down and realize that I wasn't wearing any shoes, so I would run back up the stairs only to stand there and, due to my memory deficiencies, forget why I had gone upstairs. I would then run down the stairs, go outside, and see the frost... and the whole scenario would go on and on, until something finally kicked in and I would put shoes on.

At the time I had wonderful next-door neighbors who sat on their enclosed porch and drank their coffee in the morning. They saw me running in and out of the house, up and down the stairs. I was their morning circus. One day they invited me over for dessert. They made beautiful pies, ice cream, and berries to share. When I went to their house, my neighbor asked me if I had ever been in an accident.

He said he had noticed me running in and out of the house every morning, and it seemed as if something was wrong. I couldn't believe it. I had been doing such a good job of concealing what I was going through—at least I *thought* I had—and he had seen right through it. I was stunned, but I answered honestly and told him that I had two head injuries from car accidents. Moments later his wife came out onto the porch with three books on the brain. They said they wanted me to have the books and hoped they would prove helpful to me.

I was grateful to my neighbors, but I put the books on my desk and didn't touch them for a while. Although my symptoms were an ongoing issue, I was functioning just fine at work. I was determined to succeed and took very seriously my responsibility to be on top of my game for the benefit of the children who looked up to me. I had to be their role model as well as their teacher. I wanted to see them succeed as well. My students were an antidote for me; they brought me joy that I wasn't feeling anywhere else in my life. I was in survival mode, trying desperately to live normally when there was nothing normal about what I was going through.

Long-term memory loss was another symptom that took me a while to discover. You don't realize what's missing—or how much is missing—until you are required to recall something that is no longer there.

I do not recall any of my life experiences prior to the age of twenty. I have recovered some minor incidents that occurred very close to the time of the first accident, but aside from that I have no recollection of my life prior to the accidents. I discovered this by interacting with family members, when stories would come up and I would be completely blank. They would prompt me by saying, "You know, you were there. Don't you remember?" But I really didn't remember. I had no connection to any of the events they mentioned. I would look at pictures with the hope that they would jog my memory, but again, nothing would come. The switch had been turned off and didn't appear to be coming back on anytime soon. This left me feeling lost in time. I had no recollection of where I had come from and was simply surviving each day with no emotional connection to people, places, and things I knew prior to age twenty.

Emotionally, I was blank and disconnected. To this day I have not recovered the long-term memories, although I am able to currently participate in conversations about my life prior to age twenty because of my family's efforts to teach me about my life. My family has shared many of my life experiences and events with me, but these are not stored in my brain as a personal memory. These experiences and events that they have shared with me are now stored as new information, so I am able to access the information, but I can't feel it the way someone feels a memory. There isn't any visual recognition or emotional connection to the information.

The long-term memory loss was particularly troubling for family members because my Dad passed away when I was fifteen years old. I had come home from school one day and my Mom and I had found he had passed quietly in his sleep from a heart attack at forty-four years old. This is one of the traumatic memories that was erased with my head injuries. I consider it a blessing to not have access to that particular memory, but it was confusing for some time to realize that I didn't know my Dad. I couldn't remember him at all and still cannot access the file in my brain that holds memories of him. However, through the efforts of my family I have learned about him and developed a relationship with him in spirit because I do believe he continues to watch over me, regardless of my memory loss. I also tend to think that the things I see in each of my brothers and sister are reflections of what he must have been like, especially in their sense of humor.

Memories can be a blessing and a curse for many people. Memories act as bridges to different times in our lives, but they also act as bridges between people. The long-term memory loss had become more of a burden to those around me who wanted so much for me to remember so that we could feel the bridge between us, but for me I was just blank. There was no connection. There was no bridge. I didn't know what was missing until it was brought to my attention that something wasn't there any longer. During this journey, I discovered that I was not carrying the burdens that many other people were carrying. I didn't have any bridges or connections to the past. I had a clean slate. There was a short period of time of approximately four to five months where I recognized that I had been given a "freedom" that other people around me did not have. I was not carrying burdens of the past because of my memory loss. This period of excitement and realization did not last for very long, as the realization and education that there was real damage in my brain began to set in.

CHAPTER 4

SYMPTOM SPECIFICS

A myriad of cognitive-function issues and emotional-function issues go hand in hand with a traumatic brain injury (TBI). These symptoms are probably the most confusing for someone living with a TBI because you feel that you have little or no control over them. Because the brain can regenerate, my motor skills improved over time, my vision cleared, and my problems with sensing temperature subsided, but I was left with different kinds of issues that weren't so easily cleared up. Some of the cognitive-function issues that I experienced were difficulty being understood, difficulty communicating, and difficulty understanding others. All of these symptoms involve communication, but to me they were different from each other. Let me explain how.

I often felt like people were not understanding me. I had so many clear and valid thoughts, but because I had some language-processing issues, sometimes I would get tongue-tied, or I would stutter, or—my personal favorite—I would flip syllables. The syllable flipping was terribly embarrassing because my words came out sounding like nonsense or gibberish. I often got blank stares from people because they had no idea what I was saying or even trying to say.

On the other hand, difficulty communicating meant that I had a hard time getting my point across. Even if I spoke in clear words and sentences, I often felt like I wasn't sending the right message. It was as if I were trapped inside my body and saying, "Please, someone listen! Someone hear me."

Finally, I had difficulty understanding others because I couldn't follow and decode their language quickly enough. This is where working with children was a blessing for me, because teaching beginner music involved breaking everything down to the simplest level. Concepts made sense to me at that basic level, but anything more complex was too hard for me to process. When most people speak, they don't think about "dumbing down" their language, for lack of a more appropriate way to say it. I listened to people intently yet often wished they would speak more slowly.

During many conversations, my friends would ask me if I was listening or if something was distracting me. "Well, yes, I'm distracted," I would think, "because I'm still stuck on your first word. It's going to take me a while to get to your five hundredth." This is precisely where my emotional-function issues cropped up. When you are living in a state of constant survival, just trying to get the everyday rhythm of your life going, your emotional needs aren't getting met. My emotions were no longer wired the way other peoples were. I was blank, aloof, and dedicated purely to trying to process information. My difficulties with being understood, communicating, and understanding others led to anger, frustration, and crying spells. It felt hopeless. I didn't believe that life was supposed to be about simple survival, yet that's all I felt like I was doing every day.

The crying spells were deep, soulful, sobbing cries of desperation that nothing and no one could console. I can't even tell you what the crying was about or what prompted it—perhaps the sheer exhaustion of just surviving. I also felt a deep sadness that seemed to ring inside me like a bell, radiating to every cell in my body. It was a sense of hopelessness that I would never get better. This led to loneliness: how can you deal with others being around when you can't even connect with yourself? Loneliness is characterized by a yearning for others, but I also had a desire to be alone.

These are just a few of the emotional and cognitive contradictions that take place when you have a TBI. A tug-of-war happens inside you. You want people to be there for you, but as soon as they step in, you push them away because they get too close or they trigger something that makes you recognize a symptom that you didn't want exposed. There is also a deep sense of yearning. I believe that this comes from feeling as if those files truly do still exist within your brain, but you can't seem to access them. You yearn for what's not there as well as what you believe *should* be there.

It's a constant feeling that there is some part of you that you should know, some place you are supposed to be, something that you are supposed to be doing, some person that you wish you hadn't forgotten... and the list goes on. The combination of these symptoms with physical and mental exhaustion leads to a tug-of-war of restlessness, agitation, and extreme fatigue. The daily struggle tires you out, but when you sleep at night you are so agitated that you aren't truly resting. Nothing is being restored because you are both exhausted and somehow completely agitated. This seemingly impossible state creates extreme tension and anxiety.

For me, the most bewildering symptom was the sense of guilt that came over me. I had not had any control over the car accidents. I could not have feasibly prevented or changed them in any way.

So why was I feeling guilty? Where does this guilt come from? I suspect that this type of guilt comes from our ego. Our ego tells us that we should have had some kind of superhuman ability to alter the circumstances and outcome of an event, even if we were not at fault for it. Guilt is very difficult to overcome because it traps you inside of yourself, and you are no longer able to remember who you are at your core.

CHAPTER 5

OVERCOMING OBSTACLES

Now that I've given you a laundry list of symptoms, you might be wondering how I overcame them. The answer to that question begins with the books that my neighbor gave me—the books that I left sitting on my desk. I opened the books and read them in very small increments. It was a lot to understand, especially since my reading comprehension was impaired. I had to read parts of the text over and over again, but the turning point came when I stumbled upon the idea that the brain can regenerate. After thinking about this idea at length, I decided to try to speed up the regeneration process in my own brain. I began to realize that it wasn't normal to be angry every day. It wasn't normal to feel exhausted and bruised to the bone every night. It wasn't normal to simply survive. There had to be more to life than this.

I took each of my symptoms, one at a time, and looked it up online. Sometimes I found information that I was sorry I had found, because it was frightening to realize that I could have brain damage. I had never thought of myself as brain damaged; I had simply had a car accident. But as time went on I began to understand that even though I didn't recall hitting my head, I had had a brain injury, and maybe there was some damage up there. I contacted the brain-injury association in my state, and the staff members were very kind to me. They set me up with a free mentor, who called me weekly for several months. She helped me to see my experiences in a slightly different light and told me that in order to get better, I had to develop tools.

One of the greatest tools I developed came not from me, but from a dear student of mine. One day I was at the college that I had attended and saw a flyer on the bulletin board in the downstairs lounge of the music building that housed the practice rooms and rehearsal halls. It was a mom looking for twenty minutes of music (potentially) piano lessons for her son who had autism. I thought, "Gosh, I can do that," so I called her. She asked me to do a trial lesson with her son, and so I did. He had a blankness in his eyes and definitely didn't trust me at first. He ran right out of the room within the first minute that I was with him. I felt as if his mother thought I would quit right then, but I asked her to bring him back up to the room. Over time he sat in the corner and listened to me play some basic songs on the piano. It was good practice for me, and, well, he stayed in the room, so that was a success. Eventually he came and sat near me. The day that I knew I had gained his trust, however, was when I was sitting next to him playing a song and he put his hand on top of mine. I felt an instant understanding of trust that I hadn't felt earlier. My student often didn't connect with ideas when I put them in black and white, but I discovered that he responded quickly to color. We created his very own personalized color code for the notes on the piano. I used his color code to create songs in colored blocks. Before I knew it, he was not only remembering the colors, but also reading my color blocks and playing songs that everybody would know. A siren went off in my head, and I thought that if my student could remember things by color, maybe I could too. This is where the color-coding of my life began. I put color-coded sticky notes everywhere in my house. If it was color-coded, I could get it done.

This new strategy led to my not wanting people in my apartment because the sticky notes looked neurotic and strange, but it kept me on task. My music student taught me a lot about meeting myself where I was. He perceived the world differently from others, but so did I.

The brain is the central processing unit for our bodies and emotions. It perceives an incredible amount of information from day to day and has a myriad of ways of decoding it. When I began to research symptoms of TBI, I suddenly became aware of how I was processing information. My mother had helped me develop a tool for paying my bills because I wanted to be able to function on my own. Nevertheless, one day I received a phone call from a creditor saying that I had not paid my bill. Now, I had the bill marked, the date, check number, and amount written down in my notebook, color-coded, and logged in to the system my mother had helped me develop. There wasn't a chance I hadn't paid that bill. The creditor became frustrated with me and said, "We don't know what happened to the check. We didn't receive it. You have to pay us." I became angry. In my mind the creditor wasn't just saying that I hadn't paid my bill; she was saying that I had failed, that I hadn't remembered something correctly, that I hadn't functioned the way I thought I had. About a week later, I was talking on the phone with a friend and attempting to make something to eat at the same time. I opened the toaster oven, and what do you think I found? The envelopes for my bills, signed, sealed, and stamped. Clearly, my postman had never checked my "mailbox"! (It's okay, you can chuckle. I've learned to have a sense of humor about some of this.) This discovery meant that the creditor had been right: I hadn't paid my bill. But the bigger question was, why had it happened? The answer lay in the way my brain was processing information. The brain-science perspective taught me to look at what my brain was recognizing. A standard mailbox opens from top to bottom, and so does a toaster oven. In signaling me to put my bills in the toaster oven, my brain recognized the correct movement but did not associate the proper vocabulary with the movement. Many similar instances occurred during my recovery. Another example is when I arrived home from work and went to the kitchen to get a plate. I opened the cabinet and found a bowl of meatballs next to the plates. I was always stunned to find these kinds of things; I was clearly the culprit, yet I had no recollection of ever doing it. This was another case of my brain processing the correct movement but associating it with the incorrect object. Both the refrigerator door and the cabinet opened from left to right, but because my sense of temperature was still not working properly, my brain did not recognize that the interior of the cabinet was not cold. To this very day, my cousin who had come to stay with me during this time of discovery in my life, remembers seeing notes in the pantry reminding me that milk does not go in the pantry because it is not cold in there.

In regard to brain function, one more scenario stands out. I drank a glass of milk and got sick from it. It turns out that the milk had expired by quite a long time, but because my senses of taste and smell were not functioning fully, I didn't recognize that the milk was sour, and because I had memory deficiencies, I did not remember to check the expiration date.

This incident led me to develop a tool for checking expiration dates on food. I used a marker to write the expiration dates on all the containers in my refrigerator. On the refrigerator door I posted a reminder to check the expiration date every time I took something out. Each time one of these mix-ups took place, I went searching for answers. As I became more aware of the way my brain was operating, I developed more tools—and more tools meant living a more normal life.

These tools helped me to learn how to order and organize my thoughts and my daily activities. As I mentioned previously, knowing what to do when I woke up in the morning was a deficiency for me. As I learned to develop tools for living, I began to create color-coded checklists for each set of daily activities. For example, I would keep a picture frame next to my bed with a list of color daily activities placed inside the glass. The list inside the picture frame was the first thing that I would see when I woke up in the morning.

Activities that must take place first and foremost were in red.

1. Make the bed.
2. Open the shades
3. Locate your clothes for the day.
4. Go to the bathroom.
5. Take clothes with you to the bathroom.

After the activities on the list in the bedroom were completed, there was another strategically placed picture frame with another color-coded list of activities that needed to take place in the bathroom.

This picture frame had another set of daily tasks.

1. Wash your face.
2. Brush your teeth.
3. Turn off faucet.
4. Flush the toilet.

5. Take a shower
6. Use Shampoo. (If the hair was wet, my brain thought it was already clean.)
7. Use soap.
8. Turn off the water. (Leaving water running was always a bewildering problem.)
9. Put on deodorant.
10. Put on socks and undergarments.
11. Put on clothes.
12. Brush your hair.
13. Turn off the lights.
14. Go to the kitchen.

Following the tasks completed in the bathroom, were instructions to go to the kitchen. The kitchen then had whiteboards and sticky-notes with color-coded instructions on them. The instructions included what to prepare for breakfast and how to prepare it. There were also instructions for which medicine to take and how to take it, as well as, instructions for how to turn off appliances. Yes, a note was needed to tell me *how* to turn off appliances, not just that I had to turn them off. Staring at knobs, buttons, and lighted power switches was bewildering to me. I had difficulty understanding what the power light being on meant. *Did the light being on mean that the appliance was off or did it mean that it was on?* The confusion of this triggered frustration, impatience, and anger. There were many occasions where I did not turn an appliance off correctly. I would come home from work to find the coffee maker turned on, or worse the stove turned on. It was a frightening safety hazard that I had to learn how to correct.

These frightening instances of appliances not being correctly turn off led me to receiving thoughtful gifts from my Mom. These thoughtful gifts included coffee makers, irons, lamps, and other such items that were equipped with automatic shut-off features. I no longer had to worry about appliances being accidentally left on during the day.

Returning home at the end of each day was one of the most defeating times of the day because I felt the success of having made it through a single day, but often came home to find yet another recognition of failure. Failure many times looked like lights left on, appliances left on, and a variety of items left in strange places.

I would then begin my evening ritual of going for a walk and often wondering what other people do with their time. I had no interests. I had no connection. I didn't understand the friends I had. I was lost in time because I was unable to feel the concept of time. I was not able to discern one day from the next. It was a constant state of survival and I was missing out on truly "living". It felt like there were so many hours in a day to fill. Not only could I not possibly find anyway to fill those hours, but I couldn't feel them. Describing this phenomenon is one of the most challenging things for me. It is hard to describe what it feels like to not "feel" time. I do not have an answer to this day as to why the concept of time was not being processed properly in my brain. Although the concept of time appears to be more regulated now, *fourteen years later,* I believe the reason I don't experience it in that way anymore, is because I have developed new pathways, new interests, new memories, and new relationships. The most important of those new pathways was developing and recognizing who I am now. I have created a connection to myself, my new memories, and my new interests. These important connections help me to "feel" time by giving me a sense of past, present, and future, which is not something I had prior in the discovery of the symptoms of my head injuries.

CHAPTER 6

SEEKING HELP

As I have learned is the case with some of the soldiers, I was against undergoing any type of counseling. Reaching out to the brain-injury association in my state was a big step, but it didn't involve counseling. Family members and even friends had urged me to seek help, but it was a step I was unwilling to take. I was determined to recover on my own. Well, that changed after I moved in to a new apartment. One day I was ironing my clothes and watching a talk show on television.

The show had a panel of people who had been through different types of trauma: a soldier, a person who had been in a car accident, a person who had been in a natural disaster, and a person who had been physically abused. All of the panel members had been receiving a treatment called EMDR (eye movement desensitization and reprocessing) therapy. Even to this day I do not know exactly what it is or how it works, but I do know a soldier and a civilian who have used it with great success.

When I saw this on the television, I thought, "That's what I need. I need somebody to turn this chaos off by messing with my eyes." So I cracked open the phone book and called three counselors. Somehow this therapy seemed different from traditional counseling. It seemed less invasive and less like admitting I might be crazy or weak. Two of the counselors I called spoke to me as if I were a number. They seemed to have a standard script for taking new clients. Their lack of human warmth turned me off.

I thought, "Oh, great, I finally take a step, and this is what it's going to be like?"

Then the third counselor called me back. With great kindness, she said, "Can you please tell me over the phone what happened to you?" I shared a brief synopsis of my accidents, and she replied, "I'm so sorry that happened to you. Why don't you come in for a trial appointment, and we'll see if we are a good fit?" With that, this counselor opened the door for me to finally share what had happened to me. She did not do EMDR therapy on me. Instead, she said I needed to face the trauma and create new neural pathways in my brain. Before we could do that, though, we had to find out what was actually happening in my brain. She instructed me to return to my primary-care doctor and request that some tests be run.

I was then referred to a neurologist for a single-photon emission computed tomography (SPECT) scan, a cognitive-functioning IQ test, and an electroencephalogram (EEG). Each of these tests was emotionally challenging for me because it meant that I was going to find out for sure if I had brain damage. As it turns out, the tests showed scar tissue in the frontal and occipital lobes—the front and back of my brain.

The EEG was the most difficult test for me because I had to live with hundreds of wires and electrodes on my head for three days. When you have an injury that can't be seen, the first time you look in the mirror and see evidence of the injury with your very own eyes is overwhelming, disturbing, and heart wrenching. I think I cried for the whole three days.

I was finally connecting with a physiological injury—not a weakness, not a failure to achieve, not a lack of success, but a physiological injury that had caused so much pain. I wasn't crazy. I wasn't incapable. I wasn't stupid. I was injured, and here was the proof. It didn't matter that I didn't remember hitting my head. The way the damage was described to me is that if you are traveling at 70 miles an hour and are forced to a sudden stop, your brain travels toward the front of your skull at 70 miles an hour and makes impact. Then, when your head goes back, as in a whiplash situation, your brain hits the back of your skull and makes impact at virtually the same speed. This is why there was damage in both the front and the back of my brain. If you look at a diagram of the brain and its functions, you can see that the frontal lobe deals with executive functioning, such as concentration, planning, and focus—precisely some of my areas of difficulty. At the back of the brain is the occipital lobe, which deals with the visual recognition of objects. This is consistent with my stories about the toaster oven and the refrigerator. I was recognizing movement but not objects. The accidents had affected other areas of my brain, but those were the two with scar tissue. The parietal lobe, which is just above the occipital lobe, is where the understanding and forming of words are processed. Now, I'm not a doctor, a counselor, or a neurologist— just a public school music teacher who worked very hard to understand what her counselor and doctors were telling her. But it was this knowledge that gave me the ability to understand the process of my own recovery. It also gave me the power to succeed.

CHAPTER 7

MY GREATEST TEACHERS

Right around the time that I began counseling, I stumbled upon some volunteer work with the USO at the local military base. I don't know how or why I got involved, but I believe some kind of divine intervention led me to find something important there. The autumn of 2005 was when I began volunteering at Fort Dix and it coincided with being diagnosed with post-traumatic stress disorder from my car accidents. Along with other volunteers, I greeted flights of soldiers coming home from the Iraq War. We would line up outside of the Mobilization Readiness Battalion building and shake every soldier's hand as he or she approached the door.

I always had to fight back tears. I never wanted the soldiers to see me cry. It was an honor to be one of the first people to welcome them back to our soil.

As we greeted these flights, I could see that the eyes of some soldiers looked glazed over. I always noticed these soldiers and paid attention to how they maneuvered in the room. These were often the soldiers who ended up talking to me. We would have extended conversations that I didn't truly understand at the time. A Vietnam veteran who frequented the USO paid attention to these conversations from afar and eventually approached me. He said, "What's with you? You know something. You aren't like the other girls who come out here." I just shrugged and said, "Well, I have PTSD too." He asked me if I would join him and the other Vietnam veterans at the medical hold across the street one day a week.

The veterans would meet with the troops once a week to help boost morale for those who were wounded. I agreed to show up. Gatherings were held at the Mobilization Readiness Battalion "Charlie"

Company, which was located across the street from the building where the troops would arrive home from the Iraq War.

The first time I went, it was overwhelming. I was the only woman in the room and felt pretty small, but the soldiers always made a fuss and acted like a welcoming committee when I showed up. It felt good to be with all of them. Over time, the soldiers and I developed a sense of trust, and they became open enough to share their war stories. They would even share how they were feeling, and so much of what they were sharing matched how I was feeling, so I began to share what had happened to me.

We realized that it didn't matter that I had never been to war because I was describing the same symptoms they were. They treated me like one of them and would often tell me that I was as much a warrior as they were. I didn't quite understand that until very recently.

There was one soldier I met the first year I went to these meetings. He would come downstairs every week with a sullen, sour look on his face. He never spoke to anyone and would never take any of the food or drinks we had brought. Instead, he defiantly went to the soda machine to buy the same soda every week. I watched this go on for weeks. One week, my window of opportunity opened. He went to the soda machine, and it spit out his wrinkly dollar. After watching him get increasingly angry at the machine, I took a soda, put it in my pocket, and walked over to him. I leaned on the machine and said, "Here, take this one. It doesn't want your dollar." He looked at me, snarled, and took the soda. For a minute I was afraid that he was going to yell at me or push me out of the way, but something in me knew that he knew the line not to cross. He left the room. The next week he came down and didn't go to the soda machine. Instead, he snarled and took one of our sodas. Success! I felt like I had won him over. The next week, he took a soda but stayed in the dayroom where we gathered each week for food and sodas. He took a seat on the old blue sofa. I sat right next to him and didn't say a word. It was uncomfortable, but I felt he was a kindred spirit, and I was curious to know him. He finally looked at me and said, "What is with you?" I said, "I'm Susie. I just want to know your name."

He laughed and told me his name. I couldn't help but laugh and say how awkward it was. The following week he looked for me, and we began to talk.

He was in pain. He missed his family; it had been several months since he had seen them. He couldn't bear to hear his wife cry over the phone and not be able to make her feel better. He was sad and alone, and he didn't know how to reach out for someone who cared. We became fast friends. In time, he would call his wife while I was there with him. I spoke with her over the phone and let her know he's trying to get better; "He loves you."

I remember the day he left *Charlie* Company. We both had tears in our eyes because we had found great comfort in learning each other's stories, and it was the first time we had been truly willing to trust someone with what had happened to us. There were a number of occasions that the soldiers I spoke with did not want to share with their families, friends, and spouses what they were really going through. They couldn't possibly explain what it felt like to be suffering with invisible mental and emotional wounds that were far greater than the physical wounds. It wasn't something they knew how to put into words.

After that, more soldiers sought me out. They wanted to know what I knew, and they wanted to be the next person to get special attention from me. We even had a silly paper crown that they would wear when they sat next to me. We would laugh each week and looked forward to making light of our inequities. This was healing in action.

The soldiers have become my greatest teachers and my most loyal advocates. I can't ever know where they have been, and they can't know where I have been, but we have found common ground in the process of recovery. I learned from them that it doesn't matter what your trauma is, the process is the same, and when we separate ourselves from the judgment of what we've been through, the real healing can begin. We cannot compare our trauma to the trauma of the person next to us because trauma is so deeply personal. This is very apparent when you talk to a soldier who gets hurt on a base in Afghanistan and feels like his injury isn't worthy because he wasn't in the heat of battle. Or a soldier who is ashamed that he was injured in the United States and never deployed with his unit. These scenarios lend themselves to comparison with the trauma of people who have been in battle or who have experienced a serious crisis, but the reality is that your trauma is your trauma. It's important to get out of the business of comparing. You are where you are, and you feel as you feel. It's important to own that and to grow from it, not to imprison yourself because of it.

I have crossed paths with hundreds of soldiers with hundreds of stories, many of whom I will never forget for their kindness toward me and their compassion for my journey. They were often unsure why I was there and couldn't understand my willingness to give up my time to be with them when I had my own battle to wage in my own life. Why were they worthy of my time? Well, because they made me worthy of theirs. It was an even exchange, and it brought me safety. This safety was exactly what the counselor I had been seeing predicted would happen for me. She had said that this was going to be a very profound learning experience for me and that in supporting them, I would find my way too.

CHAPTER 8

THE PROCESS

Throughout the journey I have described, I didn't really understand the process that was unfolding. Sure, I was discovering symptoms, doing some homework, and trying to live more normally, but I didn't really look at the whole picture until recently. As the wars in Iraq and Afghanistan continued, "warrior transition units" were developed to assist soldiers returning from deployment get medical care and transition successfully back to their units or transition out of the military into civilian life. When the Warrior Transition Unit was formed at the base, it was no longer called "Charlie" Company because it no longer belonged to the Mobilization Readiness Battalion. Therefore, "Charlie" company became the Warrior Transition Unit (WTU).

In the summer of 2013, I shared my story with the commander of the Warrior Transition Unit. We instantly connected. "You are the expert on your injury," she said, and suggested that I talk to the soldiers for Brain Injury Awareness Month. This idea was exciting but scary. I had never packaged my injury into a presentation before. Months passed, and February rolled around. I contacted the commander to ask if she still wanted me to give a talk, and she said yes. I had planned to just go in and do what I've done in this book—talk and tell the story—but then I decided that I needed to bring it to life and sat down to make a PowerPoint presentation. I packaged my injury for human consumption. The presentation went very well, and at the end the commander and another non-commissioned officer presented me with a thank-you certificate.

I was stunned. Never did I think that was how the day would unfold. As they read the certificate out loud, tears welled up in my eyes. It was recognition not just of my volunteering, but also of me as a person, in a way that I had never recognized myself. I was honored. The commander asked me if I would come back to do another presentation. She said that others needed to hear my story. And so it began, I had the opportunity to give a presentation to non-commissioned officers (NCO's), followed by a presentation for officers.

Here is my recovery process in outline form, as I created it for my presentation.

Awareness: You have to recognize and acknowledge that you have a problem before you can solve a problem. Recognizing a behavior as a symptom is important. I became aware that it wasn't normal to be angry all the time. It wasn't normal to have crying spells. It wasn't normal to put my mail in the toaster oven. I had to become aware of every symptom and label it as a symptom.

Education: Once I identified something as a symptom, I had to educate myself about it.

Development of tools: The danger of educating yourself about a symptom is that you now own the responsibility of choosing to do something about it or develop a tool to work with it.

Acceptance: It's important to accept that what you've learned needs to be addressed and dealt with. Sometimes what you learn isn't what you wanted to hear.

Perseverance: Identifying one symptom, educating yourself about it, and developing a tool to address it isn't enough, because opening the door to one symptom allows others to follow. You have to stay with the process, because once you develop awareness you will begin to see more and more.

Patience??: Why question marks? Question marks are here because I didn't have any patience with myself. I wanted someone to press the off switch and make all of my struggles go away, but I have learned over time to be more patient and compassionate with myself.

Attention: It's important to pay attention to how you are evolving. Paying attention to the things that are improving is just as important as paying attention to the symptoms that are plaguing you. If you only ever give attention to the negative, the positive doesn't have a chance to flourish.

CHAPTER 9

FEAR AS FUEL

We have begun to hear more and more about post-traumatic stress disorder (PTSD) as it relates to soldiers coming back from war. Scientists are doing a lot of research on it, and people in all walks of life are desperately trying to wrap their minds around it. I'm not going to talk too much about this disorder because it would require its own book, but I want to mention some co-occurring symptoms that happen with TBI and PTSD. Fatigue, depression, irritability, agitation, anxiety, and frustration are just some of the symptoms that go hand in hand with both conditions.

Specifically, PTSD involves re-experiencing a traumatic event. I suffered from flashbacks and night terrors due to PTSD, but the part that I find both fascinating and bewildering is that TBI masked these symptoms for quite some time. In the beginning of my recovery the TBI symptoms were more apparent, largely because they affected my daily functioning. These symptoms were more concrete, and I could make sense of them by understanding the physiological changes to my brain.

On the other hand, the flashbacks and the emotional trauma associated with PTSD are not so easily explained. They are very frightening, all-consuming experiences in which the entire body reacts and the mind believes the traumatic event is happening again in that exact moment. Not everyone who develops PTSD has flashbacks as depicted many times in movies; For service members that do get flashbacks, imagine the kinds of scenarios they are re-experiencing. They can be very intense. I once met a soldier who had been in a fire. The other soldiers had told me about him. They asked me to share my flashbacks with him because he was suffering and they didn't know how to help support him. They thought if I shared what I was personally experiencing in regard to flashbacks, it might offer him some perspective.

They reported that he was too fragile and anxious ever to come into the dayroom, so they wanted me to meet him in the hallway. We set up a system whereby the soldier would wave his hand in the doorway when he arrived and I would meet him in the hallway. He told me about the fire he was in and said that he often saw fireballs coming at him—when he opened his eyes in the morning, when he entered the hallway, and whenever he opened a door. I asked the soldier, "What would happen if the fireball hit you?" Very puzzled, he looked at me and said, "It's not real." I smiled at him and said, "You're right. It's not real. But your brain believes it is." I told him that I had similar types of flashbacks—albeit unrelated to fire—and I had to stand there and let them hit me in order to take their power away. I asked him if he could summon the courage to stand there and allow the fireball to hit him, knowing that it doesn't hold the power to burn him. I predicted that the fireballs would just pass through him and disappear on the other side.

He looked at me wide-eyed, dried his tears, and asked if he could hug me. He said, "You're the only one that has made any sense of this for me." These images were real to him because the brain was convinced the event was happening right now, in this very moment. Reality spoke otherwise. There was no fire in that moment, but when you are experiencing a re-experiencing event, as in the case of PTSD, the images and sensations are about as real as they possibly could be.

I said in response to him, "That's because I've lived it." If we feed the fears inside of us, I said, the monster gets bigger. I think that is one of the biggest issues I faced with PTSD. The more you fear the images, the bigger and stronger they get. It's as if fear is their fuel. The brain has to be trained to be in the here and now, otherwise it gets lost in time with PTSD.

I can remember being in a grocery store one evening in the canned food aisle. I had been tired that day and grocery shopping was always an overwhelming task for me. Grocery stores were crowded, noisy, and confusing. Much like the soldier who could not handle the crowd of people and talking in the dayroom, my brain was not equipped to handle the chaos of information, noise, energy, and people in a grocery store.

I had been in the canned foods aisle when there had been a loud noise. I can remember flinching from the sound and having a terrible vision come over me. I felt the panic set in and dropped what I had in my hands. In feeling this sense of panic come over me, I instinctively grabbed the shelf next to me. I can remember feeling the shelf being cold. I was scared by the images I was seeing, but I can remember a thought going through my head that the shelf felt cold. In a moment or two, I realized where I was and became embarrassed by my panic. I left my cart and items in the aisle and left the grocery store without any food. I remember sitting in the car and becoming overwhelmed with tears. "Why was this happening to me?" It was like I was constantly being caught off guard. I never knew when something would trigger this startle response. "Would it always be like this for me?"

When an event like this would happen, I would always call my Mom to tell her what happened. She was good at keeping track of patterns. I had told her that I could feel the cold shelf. I kept questioning why I was able to feel the cold so strongly and clearly during an episode where my brain was clearly in another place and time.

I didn't get an answer to my query for quite some time, but I did find that whenever the sense of panic or the images came over me, I reached for something cold. My brain was remembering this experience and sensation of cold. I would put my hands on the ceramic bowl of the bathroom sink or run cold water over my hands. Sometimes I would grab an ice cube out of my glass or put my hand outside of the window of my car. Any item that offered me the sensation of cold seemed to have an impact on what I was experiencing. "Why?"

The way I have come to understand it, is this. During my re-experiencing events, my brain was locked into the past. It was trying to process what had happened to me, but my fear raged against it. I was fighting it with everything that I had in me, because I couldn't face it. It was far too upsetting, so my body and mind took on the trauma of it over and over again.

When I grabbed something cold, I created a major shift in my reality. I opened a pathway in the brain that made it recognize what was happening right now. The current event was not the image I was seeing. The cold item was what was real.

Using this method of grabbing something cold whenever I had a re-experiencing event helped anchor me to the present moment, much like I have learned to do through training the brain with meditation. While my brain was exploring and processing the past, I helped my body to become less afraid by encouraging it to recognize the safety of the present moment. The images have far less power over us when we begin to recognize that it is our fear of them that gives them their fuel.

Over time the re-experiencing episodes began to last for less time because I was training a new pathway in my brain. I was becoming less afraid of the images because I was readily able to recognize that they weren't real. I had developed a simple, useful tool that allowed me to let the images "hit" me, knowing that I was never in any danger. The images and sensations would then pass and I was left confused, but unharmed.

CHAPTER 10

DEALING WITH FEARS AND CHANGED RELATIONSHIPS

Many questions come up when you have an injury, seen or unseen. You wonder if you will ever recover; will things always be the way they are now? In addition to questioning whether you will ever be normal again, you question what normal *is*. When you have an injury that can't be seen, others cannot tell that your normal is very different from them. It can take quite of bit of internal wrestling to come to terms with that.

I had a lot of questions about my memory loss. For a long time I wondered if the memories I had prior to age twenty would ever come back. If the brain can regenerate, I mused, then could my memories regenerate? Over time, I let that go.

I stopped worrying about what wasn't there and learned to embrace what *was* there. As I let go of that question, I ended up with a different question: what if the memories do come back, and they disrupt my life? What will happen to me then?

The neural pathways in my brain were shaken up, and I don't believe that so many broken puzzle pieces could ever get put back together again in one fell swoop, so I've learned not to dwell on that possibility either—although it would make for a great movie one day. In some of my conversations with the soldiers we have questioned whether we will ever be able to function like other people do. I don't think it matters anymore. We will function like who we are, not like others' expectations of us.

The soldiers and I have asked, "What if I can't ever remember who I am?" I don't think this matters either. I believe that we are evolving into who we were always meant to be, not who we think we were meant to be. Maybe our trauma is part of our evolution as a human being, not the breaking down of a human being.

We have also asked, "What will the future hold for me?" I don't know, but I sure am excited to find out, because the soldiers have shown me the very best of who I am. When I walk into the room, they do not see a broken person. They do not see a blinking beacon that says PTSD AND TBI over my head. They see grace, beauty, compassion, light, radiance, and wisdom. I know this because many of the soldiers have very sincerely told me not to hold any of these qualities back, but to embrace them and to share my story with others because they believe I can help.

I do experience a sense of loss when it comes to connections and relationships with others. To this day, other people sometimes say it's hard to read me and sometimes take offense at how aloof I seem. But my brain is no longer wired—as theirs are— with the types of experiences that help me to shape my reactions to different events and situations. I experience many things from an objective standpoint because I do not have the emotional markers or the frame of reference that others developed while growing up. It is a bit like how a child views the world. New experiences are happening all the time and I am consistently intrigued and inspired by new places, new people, new events, and new situations. I can't say that I always understand other people's strong reactions to specific situations, but I observe them and allow myself to determine if it is a positive response they are taking or a negative reaction because a choice always exists. It helps me to continue learning about the human behavior I am simply not wired for.

When you are experiencing a struggle of this magnitude within yourself, it's very difficult to explain it to other people. I've discovered a common misconception that if you have an injury that can't be seen, or if you have PTSD without TBI, you should somehow be able to control it or turn it off. This is simply not the case. There isn't an off switch for PTSD, and although I do consider myself recovered from what I went through, I am not cured. PTSD is a lifelong condition that comes with a myriad of triggers. I do, however, believe in management of PTSD and TBI, as demonstrated by my being able to live a fairly normal, happy, fulfilling life and by having the courage to talk about it.

Many of the soldiers I meet with worry that no one will understand what they've been through or where they've been. I felt like that too, but I eventually came to the conclusion that it doesn't matter whether other people understand where I've been. I can only meet people where they are. It's just as important for people with PTSD to release judgment as it is for the people who love us to release theirs. We can't judge them for their lack of experience, just as we don't want to be judged by our abundance of experience. Instead, we should agree to begin a new path together—or perhaps part ways. Parting ways doesn't have to be negative; sometimes people simply grow apart because their needs are no longer being met. It's not anyone's fault; it's the nature of our evolution as human beings. A healthy relationship has to have giving and receiving, and if both are not present, the relationship can't grow. It's tough when loved ones are desperately trying to reach you, and out of fear they become angry or apply pressure. It's not that they mean to pressure you; it's just that the fear of losing you is pressuring them.

The soldiers and I have also talked about not knowing what others want us to be, or even not knowing *any* way to be. It is confusing to feel like people are pressuring you to be something other than what you are, which in turn wears down your self-esteem, because who you are now isn't good enough. It doesn't meet their criteria of what you should be. I've heard the word *changed* used in a derogatory manner on a number of occasions.

People in my life would often make comments about how I had "changed" and how I wasn't the same person anymore. I believe that we are all on a journey to our own soul, and every experience— including experiencing TBI and PTSD—brings us one step closer. The families of soldiers desperately try to keep life normal while their loved one is away, and when their soldier comes home they continue to try just as desperately. So perhaps the family members' lack of experience and lack of change are just as problematic as the soldier's abundance of experience and change. It's easy to judge either way, so it's important to release that judgment and agree to start anew together—to form new neural pathways all around. If we only feed the negative and never feed the positive within us, we stay out of balance.

When it comes to recovering from PTSD and TBI, it's important to create as many positive experiences as you can. Each time you have a positive experience, you create a neural pathway, and eventually your brain will begin to recognize those positive experiences more readily. Right now your brain relies on the negative pathways because they are what's in abundance. Begin to train the positive, and you will collect the positive. Remember when I said that the brain can regenerate? Well, this is how it happens: by training it, stimulating it, and helping it to remember.

One of the most interesting therapies the counselor worked on with me was investigating my memory through the mapping of childhood photos. She encouraged me to think like a police investigator, where I had to analyze body language, facial expressions, environment, clothing, and energy. I also had to determine what I was thinking in the photos, as well as, what the other people in the photos were thinking. I also had to determine what I thought they were going through in their life at the time of the photo, based on their age. I would bring photos depicting my life at various ages and we would lay them out on the floor. I had to put them in the order that I thought they took place and she would ask me questions about each photo. It was challenging because I was looking at photos of myself that I didn't recognize and people who were a part of my life, but I was analyzing them as an outsider. In order to move forward with a fresh perspective, I had to, at the very least, learn about where I had come from even if I couldn't physiologically remember it. Developing this very useful skill made interacting with people so much more effective for me because I was now reading and analyzing their behavior when they were right in front of me. I couldn't help but become astutely aware of monitoring body language, facial responses, and mannerisms, even if I wasn't totally absorbing the information they were actually speaking. I was simply reading what they weren't saying. Police officers do that all the time! You can see through this approach that being "changed" didn't mean being "broken". It meant that I was simply developing new ways of communicating and new ways of approaching my life. I was developing awareness.

CHAPTER 11

EXPERIENCING LIFE THROUGH NEW EYES

Experiencing life through new eyes means seeing yourself as recovered by embracing the good that has been a part of you the whole time. The good parts of you haven't been deleted just because you experienced something traumatic. The good parts are just buried beneath some dust, and as you sweep away the dust, you reveal bits of your own light little by little. I know this because I have met soldiers who believe the worst of themselves. They are convinced that they are evil, broken, bruised, angry, unlovable, ashamed, dishonest... the list goes on and on. When I look at them and talk with them, I see people who have an internal light that is filled with wisdom, knowledge, understanding beyond most people's day-to-day life, skill, kindness, courage, bravery, and oftentimes charm and a sense of humor. If we have the power to see good qualities in each other, then we also hold the power to see the good qualities in ourselves. I once said this to soldiers as part of a briefing speech at a USO welcome-home flight:

"I stand here before you representing your wives, your girlfriends, your sisters, your mothers, your families, and your children, and I am here to remind you that you are our heroes—even on the days when you look in the mirror and cannot find the hero inside yourselves."

This is what I believe. We all have goodness inside of us. It doesn't matter where we've been or what our trauma is. We matter. I matter. You matter. Embrace that you are here. Embrace that you were led to read this story, and know that your own soul is what calls out to you to pay attention. You are not here to harm yourself; you are here to heal yourself.

Here is another short outline of how to experience life through new eyes:

Learn who you are now: How do you feel about certain topics? How do you like to dress? What foods do you like? What qualities are important to you?

Foster new interests: It doesn't matter what you liked to do before. Find out what you like to do now. What intrigues you now?

Develop new skills: It's important to take your new interests and develop them, so that new skills come from these positive experiences.

Support new neural pathways: It doesn't matter if you always used to do something a certain way.

If it isn't creating a result you like, then create a new neural pathway to a result you do like.

Accept yourself: Release judgment of yourself. Accept that you've arrived and you are going to take some new steps. It's okay.

Build positive relationships: Seek out people who empower you and inspire you. They are worth their weight in gold.

The counselor had shared with me that I would cycle through the many stages of development because the brain had to "catch up" to where I am in regard to my actual number age. This meant that I would likely not physically and mentally age in quite the same way as others do; this is due to the constant flow of new experiences that would forever be a part of my life. I will always have a childlike perspective of things being new for me. Children often recognize this in me. In some ways, we embrace life in much the same way. I also do not carry the mental and emotional conditioning that many people experience from growing up either. I don't have those life experiences available to me to shape my perspective, so I am in many ways an open book, learning as I go.

A person's age is impacted positively or negatively by their mindset. I know from studying meditation that the impact of stress on the brain can have a detrimental impact on the body. By learning to experience my life through new eyes, I have been able to adopt a peaceful, centered approach that makes room for "allowance". I no longer fight the system at play within me; I've learned to work with it and to "allow" what comes. This, as I have learned, is a fundamental principle of meditation.

CHAPTER 12

A REMARKABLE COINCIDENCE

For many years I concealed my injuries and my struggles. I don't know anyone who wants to put her weaknesses on display for the world to feast on, so I kept them to myself. It was a journey I was taking for myself anyway. Back in August 2013, there was a change of command at the Warrior Transition Unit where I was volunteering. I made an effort to meet the new commander because I wanted to continue my volunteer work with the soldiers. She was a kind woman, and we instantly connected. Her spirit was full of compassion and caring. I shared some of my story with her, and she shared some of hers. This was when she asked me to speak with the troops about TBI.

A few months passed, and a colleague and I went to perform for the troops in honor of Wounded Warrior Month. It was a nice day for everyone. At one point the commander stepped out to pick up her daughter, whom she had said she wanted me to meet. When her daughter arrived, she came up to me and we chatted about how she used to go to school where I teach and how she used to play the violin. I said, "Oh, how fascinating, I am an orchestra teacher." She had kind eyes and a heart as kind as her mother's. I felt something kindred with her, but nothing was registering. A bit later she was on the other side of the room, and I looked at her and gasped. I said, "Oh, my gosh! It's you!" She had been my violin student about nine years earlier. Her mother and I had known each other.

Her mother had been a nurse at the local hospital, and I had spoken to her on a number of occasions to set up extra after-school help on the violin for her daughter. The Captain was now a nurse in the Army, as well as, the commander of the very unit I had been volunteering with for eight years at Fort Dix. Her daughter, my former violin student, was now embarking on her own path in college.

It was a remarkable coincidence that helped me to see my life through new eyes because her daughter had told me how much I inspired her as a teacher and how patient I had been with her so many years earlier during the height of my own difficulties with being injured. The experience of meeting the Captain and her daughter again helped me to embrace how far I had come in my journey of recovery and how much my recovery has the ability to help so many others.

I had been far more successful in my journey than I had been able to see for myself. This is why the commander and I felt a kindred connection. We already knew one another and had been reconnected by chance all these years later. She has become a wonderful support to me and has given me the courage to share my story in an arena that is safe, effective, and useful.

CHAPTER 13

THE CAMOUFLAGED HEART

Many of us are eager to show the darkness of what we've been through but reluctant to show our light. Our hearts are often camouflaged from the world for fear of judgment, criticism, or hurt. But I've learned that when we step beyond the self-inflicted boundaries and start believing in the hope of a better day and a life well lived, then it's okay to have been where we've been, wherever we've been. The path we were on earlier in our lives may have diverged, but that's exactly where the real journey begins. If you have experienced TBI or PTSD, you have come home to uncharted territory in your soul. Grant yourself the distinct honor of reclaiming the land within your own soul, and believe that life is meant to be lived with joy, contentment, and love.

You are not alone in your journey. PTSD and TBI have created a brotherhood and sisterhood of people who carry great wisdom to teach the strength to overcome and the meaning of true courage. When you take off the camouflage placed on your heart by traumatic experiences and begin to embrace what has happened to you as a part of your journey through life instead of a detour, something changes. It becomes okay to tell your story because there are so many others like you who can learn from you.

When you've spent the better part of the life you know concealing the pain, the heartache, the confusion, and the injuries you can't see, nor can anyone else see, it becomes very freeing and very emotional to realize you no longer have any reason to hide. There is no reason to be ashamed. No reason to feel less than credible. No reason to feel guilty.

The battle ends here. It becomes the light that other people will follow. That's a lot to take in. The world I know that was safe, was the troops. They were just like me. I was just like them. We recognized the stare in each other's eyes. We knew what it meant and it didn't matter that we didn't know where each other had been. There was comfort in knowing we were in this together. PTSD doesn't discriminate and it doesn't just come from war. You don't choose it. It chooses you and it seems to backpack alongside trauma and traumatic brain injury.

CHAPTER 14

SEEDS OF SERVICE

As a young girl of ten years old, I was part of a class project in which students in my elementary school wrote letters of support to service members who were deployed to the Middle East during the Gulf War. I do not have any memory of being a part of this class project due to my memory loss, but I do have a picture frame with photos from the service member that I wrote to. One photo includes the military aircraft C-5B Galaxy and the other photo includes a C-141B Starlifter both flown in Saudi Arabia during

Operation Desert Storm. They are dated February 15, 1991. Also included in the picture frame is a colorful post-card and a patch depicting Operation Desert Storm. I had seen the pictures on top of the old antique piano my parents had bought for me as a kid and became curious recently about the pictures. I took the frame from off of the piano and opened the back of it to find a series of hand-written notes from the service member who was my pen-pal so many years ago. His name is TSGT Shelton St. Louis, United States Air Force deployed out of McGuire Air Force Base, New Jersey.

It was a very moving experience for me to find the notes he had written to me because I wanted so much to remember this memory, but the memories are blank. I have read his words over and over again trying to jog a memory, but what's gone is gone. I did however, discover a very profound connection to his words and to our correspondence with each other.

My school hosts an assembly each year to honor veterans and their service, but to also learn from them. This year I took a moment to share with the students that I had a pen-pal that served during the Gulf War when I was their age. I showed them the photos, the patch, and the post-card that I had proudly displayed on my piano at home. I explained to them that these pictures were part of a school project that I had participated in when I was their age. My pen-pal expressed his gratitude to me for caring, keeping his spirits up, and for making things better for him by keeping in touch. I believe this experience is part of the reason and the passion I have for creating experiences, like the assembly, each year for the students I have now.

TSGT St. Louis is not someone I ever had the opportunity to meet in person, but his letters clearly resonated in my heart and had a profound impact on my life's path. I may not remember the experience of our correspondence, but the spirit of service to others is still very much alive in me. I cared about supporting our troops as a kid and it has carried into my profession as a teacher, a healer, and a citizen. I have come to realize that it does not matter that I don't have any memory of our correspondence because a seed of service to others was planted within me regardless of whether I remember it or not.

Having discovered the notes from the service member on the back of the pictures makes me often ponder if my accidents and injuries were all part of the plan for my life after all and not the deviation I thought they were. I often questioned if my accidents changed the path of my life or altered who I was meant to be.

I believe now that I can safely say, the accidents were part of the path, not a deviation from the path.

I don't know whatever came of TSGT St. Louis, but if this book ever makes it into his hands, I hope to one day be able to shake his hand and thank him. I'd like to thank him for our correspondence because it has become a very important part of the story of my life. He inspired a little girl's path and it has blossomed into something I never could have dreamed of. I have learned that my heart was always with the troops. As a ten year old girl I felt compelled to show my support for them during the Gulf War and at twenty-five years old, I reconnected with that mission during the Iraq and Afghanistan wars. I believe that through my experiences supporting the troops, I was being shown a part of myself that already existed.

It has been a very recent realization for me to connect all of this with what is taking place in my life now. I thought my interest and passion for supporting the troops was a new development in my life, but fourteen years after my injuries, I believe it was an unveiling of what was already in me.

Recognition that my injuries have become part of my path and not a deviation from my path is also important in the unfolding of my recovery and the work that I do currently, helping others to heal from their trauma. The seeds of service were planted when I was young, but the development of understanding what it's like to suffer had to be lived through my own trauma. In order to be able to understand the suffering of others through their eyes, I had to live it myself. With that I return to the very beginning of my story in which I learned the meaning of being a wounded healer.

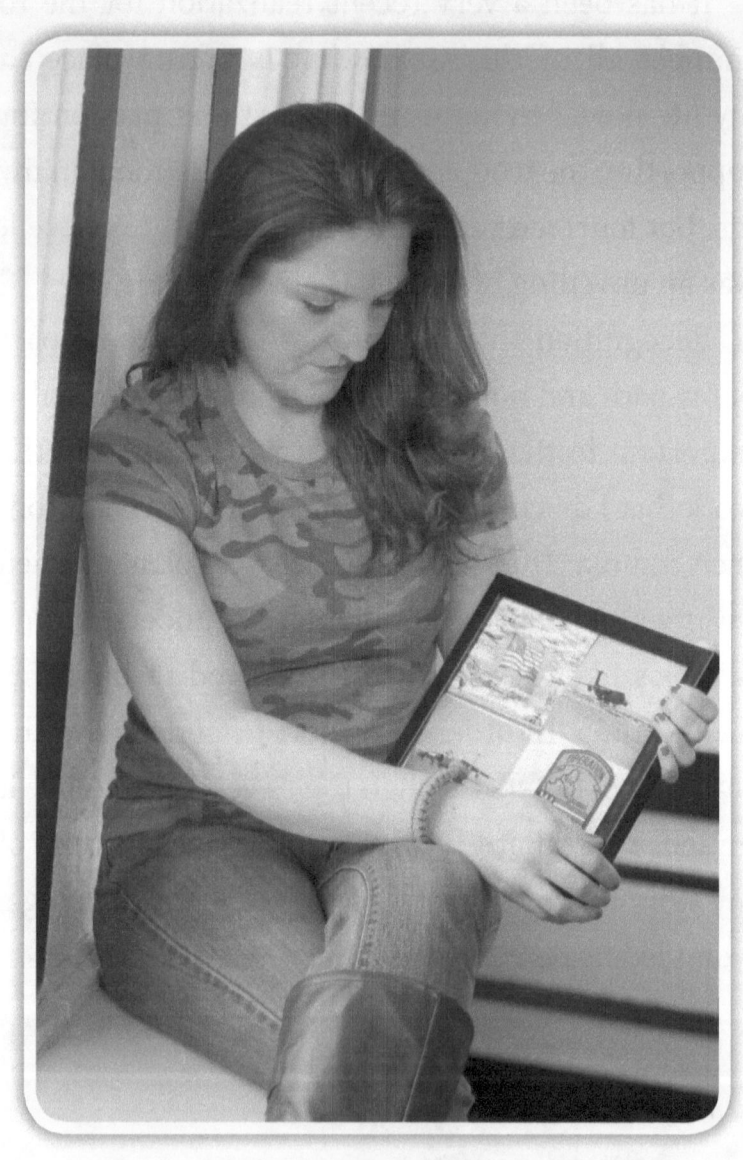

Pictures, a patch, and a postcard from my childhood pen pal during the Gulf War.

ACKNOWLEDGEMENTS

The troops of the Mobilization Readiness Battalion "B" Company and "C" Company 2005-2008: Thank you for all that you have taught me and shared with me. It will forever be my honor; *The Cadre and Staff of the Warrior Transition Unit 2013-2014:* Your kindness and bravery matters. Thank you for believing in me and for allowing me to share what I know with you and your soldiers. You granted me an opportunity and an audience to share my story; *The troops of "Charlie" Company and the Warrior Transition Unit 2005-2014:* Thank you for trusting me with your experiences and for taking me in as one of your own. I knew I was cleared as one of you when your real sense of humor came out to play. Seriousness often turned to some good old-fashioned belly-rolling laughter. Those moments were the most healing for all of us; *Michael*: For reaching out when reaching out is hard to do. If it weren't for you, I would have never stepped foot in *"Charlie"* Company. Thank you; *Bob*: Inspiration and divine intervention made us friends. You were there for our nation at 9/11 and you served our country proudly in Iraq. It is my honor to know you and call you my friend. Thank you for your encouragement, your light, and your humor; *Ken*: Amazing energy, my friend! Never mistake a light behind someone's eyes. There is always something to be learned there; *Santos*: There is nothing cooler than a saxophone-playing soldier! Thank you for giving me the opportunity to bring music into the WTU. *Miss Judy*: The lighthouse was lit but nobody was home. Thank you for being a part of the path that brought me home to me. I'm so glad I was part of your path in coming home from Iraq. It makes me so happy to see you using your own healing to help other veterans and their families. Thank you for continuing to inspire all whose lives you've touched; *Captain Stone*: You may no longer be with us, but our conversations have resonated with me long after your passing. The world was indeed a safer place because of you. May you rest peacefully, knowing you made a difference. *Vince*: You always made it a point to visit with the troops suffering from PTSD at the Army hospital. They would often ask you why you took the time to visit them when you didn't even know them. God knew why you did it. May He continue to watch over you. You always encouraged me to continue supporting the troops. You told me it mattered. You always reminded me of how important my smile and my presence was for the morale of the group. Even on days when I thought I could blend into the background, you informed me that I just can't blend. I'm meant to stand out from the crowd; *Specialist K*: Compassion was always your gift, never your weakness; *Walt*: There was no mistake when you became my friend. You always knew which soldiers needed my shoulder to lean on. I'll always remember the day you asked me to teach a soldier to dance. There were smiles a mile wide in *Charlie Company* that day. *Robyn*: For your patience with allowing me to ask you the same question over and over and over again. I can safely say, "I can finally remember the answer!" *Tyler*: My student. Thank you for teaching me to see the world through new eyes. Your spirit became a beacon of hope for me. I continue to reflect on our lessons together to this very day. You taught me to look beyond someone's eyes and into the soul of who they truly are. You are a very special person. The world is a better place because of you; *The Captain and her daughter*: Thank you for being who you are. I'm so glad our lives crossed as they have; *My Photographer Tracy Harman*; Thank you for your talent and your vision. I shared my story with you and you created a concept that gives dutiful recognition to the struggle so many people face. The photo on the cover isn't just me, it's a photo of everyone who has ever suffered the peril of PTSD and TBI. It's the way so many of us view ourselves after sustaining an invisible wound. This is what it feels like. *Lauren Koba, Makeup Artist*; Thank you for revealing the light in my eyes. You do beautiful work. *Karen B.*: You helped me develop the tools to reclaim the land within my own soul. Thank you isn't nearly enough. *Brian;* For encouraging me to go on an interview to get some experience.

There has been nothing less than an abundance of experience that has followed that very day. You have always believed in me, even long before I have the memories to support it; *Rob:* Thank you for helping me to *own* my kind of normal; *My oldest brother:* I may not remember when you left for the Navy, but Mom does. She told me that I would stand at the windows in the airport and cry every time you left because I thought you weren't coming home again. I'm very proud of your service to our country; *Vicki, "My Unofficial Battle Buddy":* You always told me I was destined to do more to help the troops. I just had to start by believing in me and stand watch waiting for the doors of opportunity to open; *Marilyn:* You took me under your wing in the USO and taught me the ropes with enthusiasm and light; *LT. COL. Reilly;* Kindness and compassion were two of your finest qualities. Thank you for the many conversations. *Lugo:* Gardening was your passion and your healing. Thank you for teaching me what you knew. You will be forever missed, but you will continue to keep all of us bound together with your jump cord bracelets; *My brother and sister;* Thank you for filling in the gaps with lots of love, laughs, and new memories. There's no denying we are definitely related! *Mom*: Your patriotism, faith, and love is greater than anyone I know. Thank you for being the example I am proud to follow. *Dad*: I didn't do this on my own. You have been whispering in my ear every step of the way. You looked out for your troops and I will continue to look out for mine. Leave the light on for me.

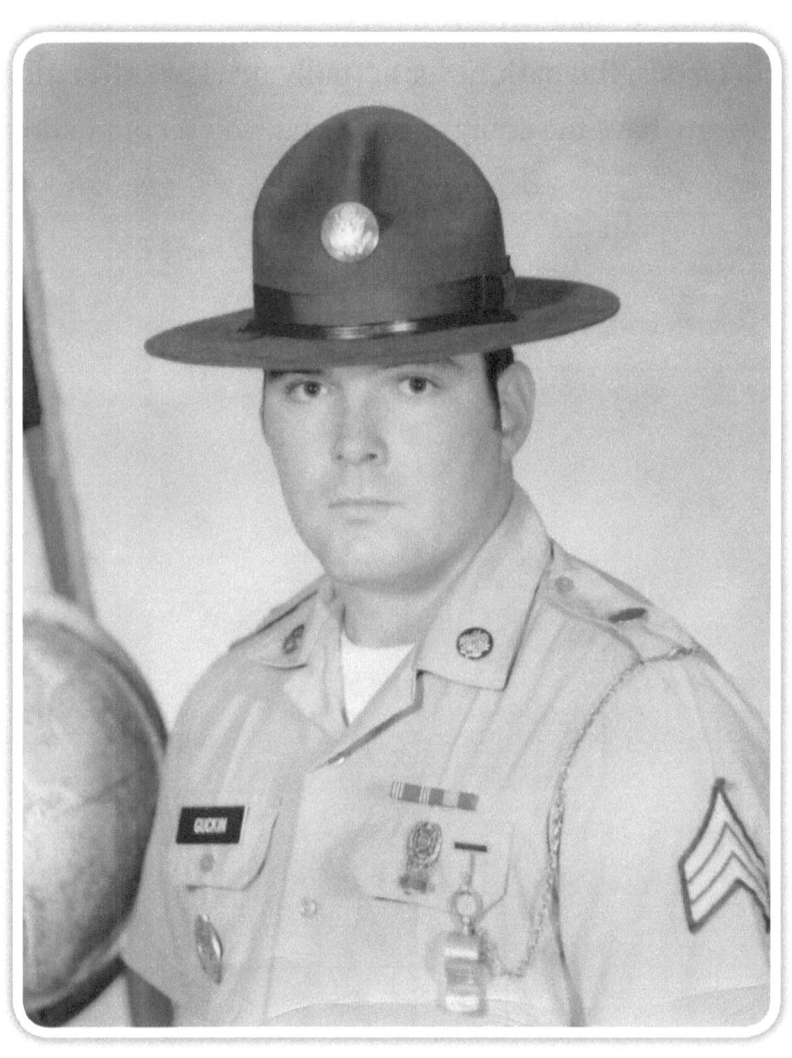

The late Sergeant Russell J. Guckin
U.S. Army Retired

To my younger self: You were far wiser than I realized. I thought that who you were had been erased. It turns out, the path never actually diverted after all. You are have me doing exactly what you set out to do.

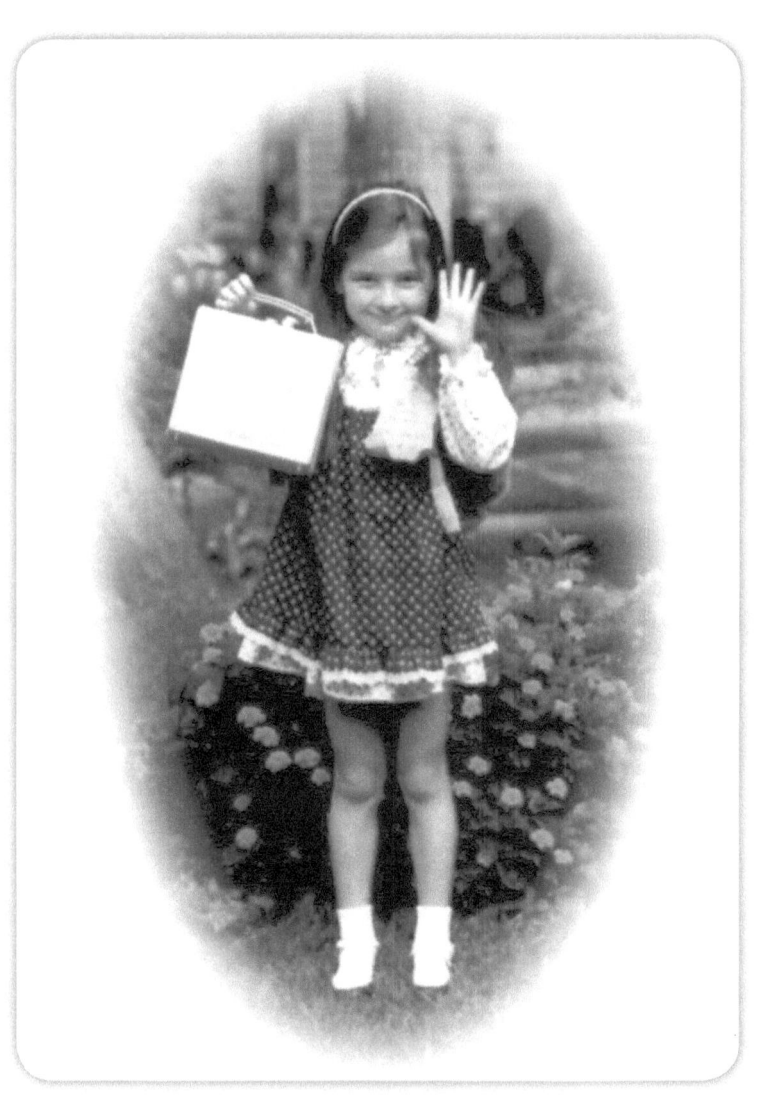

My first day of kindergarten.

Notes:

Notes:

Visit:

Peaceful Warriors
Trauma-Sensitive Meditation and Energy Work
For more information on how meditation and
energy work may be able to help you or someone
you know in their journey of recovery.

www.peacefulwarriormeditation.us